Delicious Daily Detox Cookbook

32 Taste Bud Tantalizing and Body Harmonizing Recipes

From the Creator of
foodRevelation.com

Intuitive Chef Gail Blair

Delicious Daily Detox Cookbook
By Gail Blair
Copyright 2023

The information in this book and related material in the form of tips, recipes, and nutritional guidance does not qualify as a substitution for your medical doctor's advice. Seek guidance from your doctor concerning your health and wellness, particularly with respect to any symptoms that may require diagnosis or medical attention.

First Printing 2023
ISBN: 979-8-9879358-0-4
Food Revelation
For more info or bulk ordering visit foodrevelation.com
or call 469-640-0615

Table of Contents

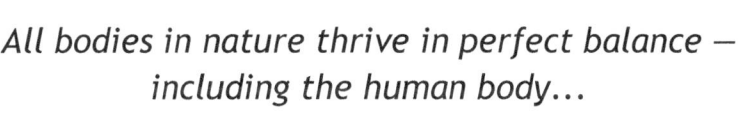

All bodies in nature thrive in perfect balance —
including the human body...

What's the Revelation?

We have been provided with the perfect tool kit for optimum maintenance and repair of our miraculous human body AND it comes from one of the greatest pleasures in life — FOOD! Glorious, Nature-made Food!

Let's face it — no one wants to suffer on the road to health. The recipes in this book are designed with everyone in mind and with one single goal — to deliver on my promise that healthy food TASTES GREAT! All it takes is a pinch of imagination and an ounce of knowledge. These recipes have been test driven to every kind of food lover, from "meat lovers" to "vegetable haters". Thank you to all my family, friends, and clients who experienced and put your stamp of approval on these recipes. The consensus is:

This is a Delicious Way to Detox!

You will enjoy these recipes long after detox. And, they are compatible with most 10-day detox programs. Choose from a variety of fantastic, simple to prepare meals, snacks, and smoothies. These recipes are easy to follow. I've even included what staple foods and tools you will need in addition to tips that will make you a rock star in the kitchen. You add the love and the food will LOVE you back!

Give your body the "clean slate" it needs to get on the right track to good health. If you are trying to nail down what foods might be causing you problems, this book naturally removes the most common allergens such as: corn, wheat, soy, dairy, eggs and all additives and preservatives. You will easily be able to determine after detox which of these foods are irritating to your body by adding them back to your diet gradually, one at a time*. Along the way you will lose your cravings for fake, processed foods and start craving, delicious, fresh, bright flavors from the good green earth.

*Want to know what foods are most compatible to your body before you begin? Go here to schedule an Intuitive Food Compatibility Session with Gail: https://www.foodrevelation.com/schedule/

> *"The Taste buds don't care if the food is plant, animal or healthy as long as it's delicious!"*

I hope you enjoy this little detox recipe book and it inspires you to fall in love all over again with food — Real Food...that not only fuels the body, but also tantalizes the taste buds.

NOTE: A body suffering from digestive distress is going to be A LOT happier with cooked foods, soups and smoothies, allowing the digestive organs to rest and repair. Be sure and drink plenty of natural spring water to help the body move out toxins.

The Well-Equipped Kitchen

Sharp Things & Such

- ✓ Sharp chef's knife for chopping, mincing, and shredding
- ✓ Serrated knife for bread & tomatoes
- ✓ Paring knife for peeling and small jobs
- ✓ Large and small wooden cutting boards (or acrylic)
- ✓ Steel for sharpening

Cutting Tips

Always cut on level, stable surface.

Place wet towel under board to prevent slippage.

Always give your chef's and paring knife a few swipes across a steel before and after use to maintain a sharp edge.

For Draining and Straining

- ✓ Large stainless colander
- ✓ Small fine mesh metal strainer
- ✓ Large fine mesh metal strainer
- ✓ Large slotted metal spoon

I like metal strainers and colanders for hot foods. Plastic can melt under high heat and end up in your food...yuk! Plastic is fine for rinsing fresh fruits and vegetables.

For Mixing & Baking

- ✓ Assorted sizes of glass and stainless bowls
- ✓ Assorted casserole dishes
- ✓ Baking sheets and glass pans

- ✓ Electric or stand mixer
- ✓ Good kitchen timer

For Stove Top

A good set of stainless or enamel coated iron cookware should include:

- ✓ Stock pot with lid
- ✓ Medium sauce pan with lid
- ✓ Small sauce pan with lid
- ✓ Large skillet with tight fitting lid
- ✓ Small skillet

In Addition

- ✓ Wooden spoons and spatulas
- ✓ Stainless or silicon tipped tongs
- ✓ Stainless and silicon spatula
- ✓ Stainless or silicon steamer basket
- ✓ *Well-seasoned iron skillets

Skillet Tips

A stainless steel skillet can be virtually non-stick if (1) you polish it regularly (I use Bon Ami) and (2) you heat it before using.

I use my old iron skillets for everything from sautéing to baking. A well-seasoned skillet never sticks. Just a few tips from my Dad on caring for iron skillets:

*Do not use soap in your skillet unless necessary. Scour (with plastic) and rinse with hot water. If you do end up burning food in your skillet do not scrape it! Fill skillet with water and heat to simmer for a few minutes. The food will come right off.

*To dry skillet thoroughly, place it over low heat or in a warm oven until completely dry. You may then rub the skillet with a small amount of vegetable oil if you do not plan to use it again soon. This will protect it from moisture. Never put oil in a damp skillet — it will lock in the moisture and cause it to rust quickly!

Never cut in your skillet with a knife. It will damage the seasoning and cause it to stick in that spot. You will have to re-season it (coat with oil and bake).

I use lemon juice and course ground salt to scour a rusty skillet. Dry very well and then coat skillet with small amount of oil, turn upside down in oven and bake at 350°F for 45 minutes. You may need to repeat until a paper towel rubbed in the skillet comes away clean. I've had to repeat this process up to 3 times. *If you follow the first 3 tips, you will never have to do this again!*

Food Prep Station

- ✓ Potato peeler
- ✓ Microplane for zesting
- ✓ Lemon/lime juicer
- ✓ Orange juicer
- ✓ Assorted glass or stainless bowls
- ✓ Stainless or glass portion cups

Prep Tips

A microplane is an indispensable tool for zesting citrus, finely shredding cheese, and grating nutmeg.

Assorted size glass bowls and portion cups allow you to measure and have ready all ingredients before you start cooking. This will save you time and mistakes.

The Obvious and Not So Obvious

✓ Set of stainless steel measuring cups and spoons

✓ Small processor & large processor

✓ Extra small processor for flaxseed and to grind other seeds and spices

✓ 2 and 4 cup glass measuring cups

✓ Immersion blender

✓ Parchment paper

✓ Assorted glass storage containers with lids (like Pyrex or Ball jars)

✓ Assorted plastic freezer bags

✓ Good pepper grinder — nothing beats fresh cracked pepper

You do not have to have a processor, but they sure do make your life easier. I have a small and large Cuisinart. The small one is perfect for making hummus and chopping garlic and hot peppers. I received as a gift a "Bullet" blender. What a great tool for making quick smoothies and dressings. The immersion blender also saves you the hassle of transferring hot soups to a processor for pureeing. Simply "immerse" the blender in the pan and turn it on. A great, handy invention — wish it was mine! Of course, you can use an old fashioned blender and hand held mixer for just about anything.

Gail's Time & Health Saving Tips

- To save time, buy minced ginger and garlic in a jar.

- To save money, shop for spices, rice and lentils at Asian and Indian markets.

- Buy spices in bulk and refill your containers — saves you money and the planet. Bonus — you can try a little before buying a lot.

- To add body to any soup, just puree a few cups and pour it back into pot — a great way to make cream soups without adding extra calories and thickeners.

- Always freeze some soup for later in 2 to 4 cup portions in freezer bags or jars. Allow to cool before placing food in plastic to avoid plastic being transferred to food.

- Never put acidic foods like tomatoes and vinegar in plastic unless freezing right away.

- When roasting or boiling vegetables cut the hardest ones smaller (like beets) or they will take longer to cook.

- Avocado and sunflower oil are great for high-heat cooking and a great way to avoid unhealthy, highly refined oils. Cold pressed oils (like olive and coconut oil) have a low smoke point; use in low to medium high heat cooking or roasting.

- Keep oils and vinegars in dark lower cabinet (it's cooler close to the floor...that goes for wine too). Any oils used infrequently, should be kept in refrigerator to prevent from going rancid.

- Add lemon and sea salt or Himalayan* at the end of cooking. Salt causes food to release aromas and flavors. Add salt a little at a time and TASTE (you will use a lot less). Lemon brightens flavors.

- Vinegar and sugar balance flavors and spark the taste buds. For instance, a little apple cider vinegar will balance bitter flavors (without adding sugar). I use it in lemonade.

- Herbs added during the cooking process, mellow and blend. For a more pungent punch, add at the end. Or, as in Italian cooking — do both! Note: Dried herbs have more concentrated flavor than fresh — use half as much.

- Always rinse beans, rice, and lentils to remove dirt and some of the starch.

- Always rinse canned beans to avoid excess gas.

- Toast rice for a few minutes in hot skillet to give it a rich, nutty flavor and aroma. Adding flaxseed during cooking helps keep brown rice separate (not sticky) and adds a healthy helping of Omega 3 fatty acid.

- Toasting spices at the beginning of a recipe, adds incredible depth to the dish. The aroma fills the senses and primes the palate.

- Keep ground flaxseed in freezer to preserve healthy lignans. Even better — grind your seeds fresh as needed. Note: whole flaxseeds are indigestible to most people.

- Roasting garlic gives it a mild, mellow flavor. Garlic makes a great, natural insect repellent. Eat it every day and mosquitos and fleas will "flee". I give it to my dogs instead of harsh, dangerous d r u g s . Note: Ask your vet for safe dosages based on weight. https://www.dogsnaturallymagazine.com/garlic-for-dogs-poison-or-medicine/

- Roasting adds a rich, depth of flavor to a variety of vegetables, especially root veggies. Roast summer veggies (high water content) at 400°F for about 5-10 minutes to retain precious nutrients.

- Always wash organic and non-organic fresh fruits and vegetables very well to remove contaminates. Buy organic whenever possible, especially those foods you eat a lot of. Pay special attention to the "Dirty Dozen List". It changes periodically. https://www.ewg.org/foodnews/dirty-dozen.php

- For longest life, make sure fresh herbs and greens are dry before placing in airtight bags. They will keep up to a week in the refrigerator.

- Only wash and cut produce you plan to use in the next few days. Store produce in a "green" bag" or air-tight container for up to 1 week in the fridge.

- Did you buy more produce than you can eat? No worries, just throw it in the freezer to use in your smoothies or soups. Blanche green beans, asparagus and broccoli to retain color.

- Buy regular vegetable broth (not low sodium) for more flavor and dilute it with water by half if watching sodium intake*. Also note: After detox buy "Better that Bouillon" organic vegetable broth concentrate in a jar. It has a little soy in it, so it's off limits for detox, but this is the best tasting broth!

- Keep baked sweet potatoes or roasted sweet potato fries on hand for snacking anytime. Store up to a week in the fridge; just pop in the toaster oven for about 15 minutes to warm. Try your baked sweet potato with a dollop of unrefined coconut oil and a sprinkle of sea salt and cinnamon... yum.

- Place fruit in paper bag to ripen quickly.

- Like the T.V. chefs, prep and pre-measure all ingredients before you start cooking to save time and frustrating mistakes.

*Not all salt is created equal. Nature-made, unprocessed salts contain body nourishing minerals in perfect balance.

The Well-Stocked Pantry, Fridge & Spice Rack

The goal is to always have on hand everything you need to prepare just about anything. You should only have to shop for fresh food, to replace stock and buy the occasional random item — great time saver! It's easier to eat healthy if you have the right stuff to make food magic at your fingertips. You don't have to get it all at once. Just choose the items needed to prepare your favorite cuisine. Experiment! A cookbook is just a template. Add your own inspiration to mine.

Save a little room in your weekly budget to add 1 or 2 spices or pantry items every time you shop. Before you know it you will have a fully stocked kitchen and will be well prepared to cook something fabulous at the drop of a hat!

Pantry Staples

✓ Extra virgin olive oil

✓ Avocado oil (cold-pressed/unrefined)

✓ Coconut oil (cold-pressed/unrefined)

✓ Sunflower oil (cold-pressed/unrefined)

✓ Spray coconut oil

✓ Red wine vinegar

✓ White balsamic vinegar

✓ Aged balsamic vinegar

✓ Sherry vinegar

✓ Bragg's coconut liquid aminos

✓ Bragg's apple cider vinegar

✓ Red lentils

✓ Brown lentils

✓ Nutritional yeast (organic)

✓ Wild rice

- ✓ Brown basmati rice
- ✓ Brown rice flour
- ✓ Arrowroot
- ✓ Tapioca flour
- ✓ Quinoa (assorted colors)
- ✓ Organic liquid stevia (NOW Better Stevia is a good one)
- ✓ Kombu (dried — usually in Asian section)
- ✓ Vegetable broth in cartons (Imagine NO-chicken broth is great!)
- ✓ Organic canned coconut milk
- ✓ Vegetable protein like brown rice, hemp or pea (no sugar added)
- ✓ Green tea

In a dark, dry spot in the pantry keep:

- ✓ Assorted onions and shallots
- ✓ Potatoes/sweet potatoes
- ✓ Fresh garlic

Spice Rack

- ✓ Whole cloves
- ✓ Ground cinnamon
- ✓ Cardamom pods*
- ✓ Cumin seeds*
- ✓ Black mustard seeds*
- ✓ Ground turmeric*
- ✓ Ground coriander*
- ✓ Garam masala*
- ✓ Ground cumin*
- ✓ Curry powder*

- ✓ Ground cayenne
- ✓ Paprika
- ✓ Smoked paprika
- ✓ Red chili flakes*
- ✓ Chili powder*
- ✓ Chipotle chili powder
- ✓ White pepper
- ✓ Black peppercorns
- ✓ Sea salt (assorted)
- ✓ Pink Himalayan salt
- ✓ Garlic sea salt
- ✓ Garlic powder
- ✓ Onion powder
- ✓ Dried bay leaves
- ✓ Dried basil
- ✓ Dried curry leaves*
- ✓ Dried tarragon
- ✓ Dried thyme
- ✓ Dried oregano
- ✓ Nutmeg ball*
- ✓ Almond extract
- ✓ Pure vanilla extract**
- ✓ Pure orange extract**
- ✓ Pure lemon extract**

*Many spices are available at Indian and Asian Markets for way less! (Whole foods markets and natural grocers carry a lot of bulk spices as well)

**Food Grade essential oils like Do Terra can be used in place of extracts (a drop goes a long way!)

Fridge Staples

- ✓ Parsley
- ✓ Salad greens
- ✓ Roma tomatoes
- ✓ Kale
- ✓ Ginger root
- ✓ Lemon/limes/oranges
- ✓ Celery
- ✓ Fruit for snacking
- ✓ Fresh carrots
- ✓ Avocado (refrigerate when ripe)
- ✓ White wine for cooking (NO DRINKING during detox!)
- ✓ Thai red curry paste
- ✓ Tahini (find with nut butters)
- ✓ Flaxseed oil
- ✓ Dijon mustard

Freezer Staples

- ✓ Mixed veggies
- ✓ Mixed berries
- ✓ Mirepoix (celery, onion, bell pepper)
- ✓ Broccoli and cauliflower
- ✓ Brussel sprouts
- ✓ Ground flaxseed

Easy, Quick, Healthy Snacks

Baked Sweet Potato Chips

6-8 Servings

2 large sweet potatoes sliced very thin (use mandolin or processor if you have one)

Coconut oil spray

1. Preheat oven to 425°F. Line 2 large baking sheets with parchment.
2. Spray coconut oil on potatoes while tossing to coat evenly. Place potatoes on prepared pans in a single layer.
3. Bake for about 30 minutes switching pans half way through until slightly brown and crispy. You can turn the potatoes if you have the patience.
4. Season them with whatever your heart desires:
   - Sea salt and cracked pepper
   - Cinnamon
   - Garlic salt
   - Rosemary and sea salt (my favorite)
   - BBQ seasoning (no sugar)
   - Blackening spices
   - Smoked sea salt

Once cool and dry, you can store these little gems in zip lock bags for a week or more. You'll want to make several batches — they will not last long! A great dipper for Red Lentil Hummus! This recipe works great with beets as well.

"To snack or not to snack, that should NEVER be the question." — LE proverb

Red Lentil & Red Pepper Hummus

16 Servings

---

2 cups red lentils, prepared and drained well

1 tbsp olive oil

1 tbsp lemon juice

2 tbsp tahini

1/2 cup roast red pepper, diced

2 garlic cloves

1/2 tsp ground cumin

1/2 tsp onion powder

1/4 tsp coriander

1/2 tsp garam marsala

1/2 tsp sea salt and cracked pepper or to taste

1 tsp fresh grated ginger (optional)

2 tbsp fresh chopped cilantro (optional)

Blend all ingredients in processor or blender. Add a little water if necessary for desired consistency.

Beautiful with sweet potato chips or celery and carrot sticks. Experiment! This is mouth-watering. Time to spice up the spice cabinet!

"Did you ever stop to taste a carrot? Not just eat it, but taste it? You can't taste the beauty and energy of the earth in a 'twinkie'". — Astrid Alauda

Fresh Veggies with Sweet Chili Lime Vinaigrette

6-8 Servings

---

2 tbsp olive oil or avocado oil

1 tbsp liquid coconut aminos

1/4 tsp red chili flakes (optional)

1/2 tsp chili powder

1 tsp ground cumin

4 drops organic liquid stevia

1/2 tsp sea salt

Cracked pepper to taste

2 lbs assorted fresh cut raw vegetables (cauliflower, broccoli, carrots, etc.)

Place dressing ingredients into food processor or jar with tight lid and blend well before serving. Toss veggies in dressing or dip. Sweet and Spicy!

Cinnamon Dusted Frozen Grapes

Remove grapes from stems and rinse well. Place in single layer on sheet pan and place in freezer until frozen (about 30 minutes). Transfer to freezer bags. When ready to serve, remove from freezer. Thaw for a just few minutes and sprinkle with cinnamon before serving.

These little frozen balls will really satisfy your "sweet snacking" tooth. You will want to keep these around all summer for a cool treat anytime! Here's something to really look forward to — I don't think I've ever had anything as good as homemade coconut vanilla bean ice cream with cinnamon dusted frozen grapes mixed in. I'm not kidding! Make it sugar-free for detox.

Curry Pickled Carrots & Radishes

---

1 cup water

1 cup Bragg's apple cider vinegar

4-6 drops of organic liquid stevia

1 tbsp course ground sea salt

1 tsp black mustard seeds

6 curry leaves

2 tbsp fresh ginger, julienned (optional)

1 jalapeno, sliced with seeds (remove seeds for wimps)

1/2 pound radishes, scrubbed and thinly sliced

1/2 pound fresh carrots, scrubbed and thinly sliced

1. In large sauce pan, bring water, vinegar, stevia, salt, mustard seeds, and curry leaves to a boil. Remove from heat and set aside.
2. Stuff ginger, jalapeno, radishes, and carrots into large mouth jars. Pour in vinegar and water mix.
3. Allow to cool and store in fridge for up to 2 weeks or use canning method to store indefinitely.

This is a delicious and unique spin on the traditional pickled offerings. Try tossing them with a little olive oil and serve on top of your favorite greens, or serve as an appetizer along with hummus, olives, and pickles. Or, just eat them right out of the jar.

Delicious Daily Detox Salads

Roasted Asparagus, Red Bell Pepper & Radicchio Salad
4-6 Servings

1 tsp extra virgin olive oil

1 bunch of asparagus, washed and trimmed*

1 large radicchio head, remove core, cut into 4-6 wedges

1 red bell pepper, quartered with seeds removed

1/4 cup red onion, sliced very thin

Dash of sea salt and pepper

4 cups mixed salad greens (or herb mix)

2 tsp lemon juice

Vinaigrette:

3 tbsp aged balsamic vinegar or Bragg's apple cider vinegar

2 tbsp extra virgin olive oil

2 tsp Dijon mustard

1 small shallot, minced

1 tsp lemon juice

Sea salt and cracked pepper to taste

1. Preheat oven to 400°F. Toss asparagus, radicchio, and bell pepper in a teaspoon of olive oil and sprinkle with a little salt and pepper. Arrange in a single layer on baking sheet and bake for about 5 minutes or until asparagus is crispy tender.
2. Blend all dressing ingredients in small processor or shake well in jar with tight lid.

3. When cool enough to handle, chop asparagus and peppers into 1" pieces. Toss them and radicchio gently with vinaigrette and red onion and set aside.
4. Toss salad greens in lemon juice and a dash of salt and pepper. Arrange roasted veggies on top of dressed greens.

This vinaigrette preserves veggies. Keep veggies in the fridge and enjoy for up to a week. They get better and better. Dress your salad greens right before serving.

*Note: When trimming asparagus, bend flat end until it breaks. It will break at the tender spot.

Red Beet, Red Onion & Red Cabbage Salad

8-10 Servings

---

1 large beet, peeled and finely shredded (don't toss the beet greens*)

2 cups purple cabbage, finely shredded

2 large carrots, shredded

1/2 red onion, sliced thin

1 red apple, julienned with skin on

1/4 cup fresh chopped parsley, mint or basil (or a combo)

Dressing:

1/4 cup olive or avocado oil

1/4 cup Bragg's apple cider vinegar

1/4 cup fresh squeezed orange juice (or 1 drop orange oil)

1 tsp orange zest

2 tsp fresh ginger root, minced

1 small shallot, minced

4 drops organic liquid stevia

1/2 tsp organic sea salt and cracked pepper to taste

1. Shred beets, cabbage, and carrots in processor or by hand. Mix together in a large bowl with onions, apple and herbs.
2. Combine all dressing ingredients in processer or place in jar with tight lid and shake well. Toss beet and cabbage mixture with dressing.
3. Arrange beet and cabbage mixture on top of lemon dressed greens (see step 4 in the prior Vinaigrette recipe). Garnish with a little chopped parsley or basil.

This colorful salad, packed with beta carotene makes a complete meal when paired with brown rice or quinoa. Try it out with Indian Basmati Rice on page 53. Another salad that will keep in the fridge for up to a week.

*Sauté beet greens with a little onion and garlic in vegetable stock — delicious!

Chili Lime Cole Slaw

6-8 Servings

1/4 head red cabbage, shredded

1/4 head white cabbage, shredded

1/2 red onion, sliced very thin

1 jalapeno, chopped fine (optional)

1 apple cored, chopped fine (skin on)

2 large carrots, julienned

2 celery stalks, chopped

1/4 cup fresh chopped cilantro

Dressing:

1/4 cup Bragg's Apple Cider Vinegar

1/4 cup extra virgin olive oil

1/4 cup fresh lime juice with 1/2 tsp lime zest

4 drops organic liquid stevia

1 small shallot, minced

1 tsp Dijon mustard

1/4 tsp cumin powder

1/4 tsp garlic powder

1/4 tsp of cayenne (or to taste)

1 tsp sea salt and cracked pepper

Whisk together dressing ingredients and toss with vegetables until well combined. Allow to stand in refrigerator for a few hours before serving. Another delicious salad that will keep up to 1 week in the fridge. Did you know your taste buds can do the Samba?

"Sharing food with another human being is an intimate act that should not be indulged in lightly" — M. F. K. Fisher

Thai Curry Slaw

6-8 Servings

---

1 cup red cabbage, shredded

1 head of bok choy, shredded (or 1/2 head of white cabbage)

1 cup fresh broccoli, chopped small (stalk removed — freeze to add to soups)

1/2 cup green onions, chopped (use some of the green part as well)

1 apple, cored and chopped (skin on)

2 large carrots, julienned

1/4 cup shredded coconut (unsweetened)

1/4 cup fresh chopped cilantro or basil

Thai Curry Dressing:

1 tsp toasted sesame oil (or 2 tsp roast tahini)

1/4 cup olive or avocado oil

1/4 cup Bragg's apple cider vinegar

1 tsp lemon juice

1 tsp minced garlic

2 tsp minced ginger

1-2 tsp Thai red curry paste (to taste)

1/4 tsp curry powder (mild or hot)

4 drops organic liquid stevia

1/2 tsp sea salt

Whisk or blend together dressing ingredients and toss with vegetables until well combined. Allow to stand in refrigerator for a few hours before serving. Store for up to 1 week in fridge.

There is nothing boring about this salad. When detox is over, try it with sliced avocado on Ezekiel Sesame Seed Flourless Bread...Wild!!!

"One of the very nicest things about life is the way we must regularly stop whatever it is we are doing and devote our attention to eating" — Pavarotti, My World

Figs & Fennel Salad with Mixed Baby Greens and Kale

6-8 Servings

My all-time favorite salad! The sweetness of the figs and the tartness of the kale when combined with the fresh tantalizing orange essence — creates a perfect symphony that fills the senses.

2 cups kale, torn into small bite size pieces — stems removed

1 large fennel bulb, washed trimmed and sliced very thin

4 cups baby greens

1/4 cup red onion, sliced very thin

1/2 cup fresh figs, quartered (substitute apples or pears in season)

Orange Sherry Vinaigrette:

1/4 cup sherry vinegar

1/4 cup avocado or olive oil (add 2 tbsp of whole avocado for creamy version)

4 drops organic liquid stevia

1 drop food grade orange oil (or 2 tbsp fresh orange juice with 1 tsp zest)

1 small shallot, minced fine

1/2 tsp sea salt and cracked pepper to taste

Water for consistency

Blend dressing ingredients in a small processor or blender. Add kale and dressing to large bowl and massage with clean hands until kale is reduced by half (3-4 minutes). Add the rest of salad ingredients and toss until blended well.

Quinoa Tabbouleh

6-8 Servings

2-3 garlic cloves, minced fine

Juice from 1 large lemon

1 cup diced cucumber, peeled or unpeeled (your option)

1 cup cherry tomatoes, halved

1/4 cup finely sliced green onions

3/4 cup chopped curly parsley

3 tablespoon of extra virgin olive oil (omit for oil-free version)

1 teaspoon sea salt

Cracked black pepper to taste

3 cups cooked quinoa

In large bowl mix together everything except quinoa. Gently fold in quinoa into vegetable mix. Refrigerate for at least 1 hour. Garnish with sliced avocado before serving for added protein and healthy fat.

Note: For a spicy southern spin add a diced jalapeno and chopped avocado; replace 1/2 of parsley with fresh chopped cilantro.

"A jazz musician can improvise based on his knowledge of music. He understands how things go together. For a chef, once you have that basis, that's when cuisine is truly exciting" — Charlie Trotter

Delectable Detox Soups for EVERY DAY

Curry Red Lentil Soup

8-10 Servings

1 tbsp coconut oil

1 onion, finely chopped

2-3 garlic cloves, minced

1 tsp ginger, minced

1 tsp black mustard seeds

1 tsp ground cumin

1 tsp garam masala

1 tsp ground turmeric

1/4 tsp ground coriander

1/4 tsp cayenne (or to taste)

1 cup carrots, diced small

1 1/2 cups red lentils, rinsed well

6 cups vegetable broth

2-3 curry leaves (or 2 bay leaves)

1 bunch of Swiss chard or spinach, chopped

1 large tomato, diced

Water as needed

Sea salt to taste (a little at a time)

Cilantro for garnish

1. In large pot, melt coconut oil over medium heat. Add onion with a dash of salt and sauté gently until starting to caramelize (about 15 minutes, stirring often).
2. Add garlic, ginger and mustard seed sautéing for a couple more minutes. Add spices stirring constantly for another minute to toast.
3. Add carrots, lentils, broth, and curry leaves. Bring to simmer and cook with lid on for 20 to 30 minutes until lentils and carrots are tender. Add more water if needed.
4. Partially puree if desired. Add tomatoes and chopped greens. Re-heat gently. Garnish with fresh cilantro and diced tomato.

This fragrant Indian staple provides delicious whole protein. Serve with a colorful salad for a complete meal.

"Always start out with a larger pot than what you think you need" — Julia Child

Curried Vegetable Soup

4-6 Servings

---

1 lb of cauliflower, cut into florets

1 cup canned coconut milk

2 cups vegetable broth

1 tbsp curry powder

Dash of cayenne (or to taste)

1/2 tsp white pepper

1 cup frozen cut green beans

1 cup fresh carrots, shredded

1/4 cup fresh, chopped cilantro (reserve a few springs for garnish)

1 tsp lemon zest

Dash of nutmeg

Sea salt to taste

1. Combine cauliflower, milk, broth, and curry in large pot. Bring to boil. Reduce heat and simmer covered for about 15 minutes or until cauliflower is fork tender.
2. Add white pepper, cayenne and green beans to pot. Bring to simmer for another few minutes until beans are heated through.
3. Remove 2-3 cups of soup and puree (an immersion blender comes in handy for this). Add pureed soup back to pot with carrots, cilantro, lemon zest and nutmeg. Re-heat gently. Garnish with a sprig of cilantro and a lemon wheel before serving.

Simple comfort food and a great "pick-me-upper" anytime!

"I live on good soup, not on fine words". — Moliere

Savory Cream of Mushroom and Leek Soup

8-10 Servings

1/2 cup vegetable broth

2 large leeks, chopped with green top removed (wash well)

3-4 garlic cloves, minced

1/2 tsp fresh rosemary, chopped with stem discarded (or 1/4 tsp of dried)

1 tbsp fresh thyme, chopped with stem discarded (or 1 tsp dried)

4 cups of mushrooms (mix it up with shitake, cremini, and buttons)

3 tbsp brown rice flour or tapioca flour

1/4 cup water (or dry white wine after detox)

5 cups vegetable broth

1/2 cup of canned coconut milk (optional)

Sea Salt and cracked pepper to taste

1. In large pot heat 1/2 cup of broth over medium high heat. Add leeks and a dash of salt, sautéing for 3-5 minutes or until leeks are translucent. Add garlic, rosemary, thyme, and mushrooms. Sauté until mushrooms have released their moisture (about 5 minutes). Keep moving — do not burn herbs.
2. Sprinkle the flour over mushroom mixture, stirring a few times to blend and toast the flour (do not burn flour). Add wine (or water) to deglaze the pan, allowing alcohol to evaporate for a minute, stirring constantly.
3. Slowly add broth and stir until well blended (no lumps). Bring to simmer for a few minutes until soup is just beginning to thicken.
4. Puree 3-4 cups of soup for a smoother texture if desired. Blend in coconut milk and re-heat gently.

When you are craving something rich, creamy and savory on the palate — this soup will not disappoint!

"When I was a young man, I had a mentor on women and he said when you meet a woman that you think you like, don't ask her for a drink. Take her out for a bowl of soup. Because a woman who can enjoy a bowl of soup is bound to be more interesting" — Art Cooper

Indian Spiced Root Vegetable Soup

10-12 Servings

1/2 cup water or vegetable broth

1 large onion, chopped

2 stalks of celery, chopped

2-3 garlic cloves, chopped

1 tsp fresh minced ginger (or 1/2 tsp ground)

1 tsp ground turmeric

1 tsp ground cumin (or 1/2 tsp seeds)

1 tsp chili powder

1/2 tsp paprika

Dash of cinnamon

1/4 tsp cayenne (or to taste)

1" sprig of fresh rosemary, chopped fine, discard stem (or 1/4 tsp dried)

1 large apple, cored, peeled and chopped

2 large carrots, chopped

2 parsnips, chopped

1 medium rutabaga or turnip, peeled and cubed

1 large sweet potato, peeled and cubed

1 small golden beet, cubed small (optional)

6 cups of vegetable broth

1 bunch of Swiss chard, pulled from stems and chopped

Sea salt and cracked pepper to taste

1 cup canned coconut milk (optional)

1. Heat large soup pot over medium high and add 1/2 cup of water or broth. Toss in onion, celery and a dash of salt. Sauté about 3 minutes until onions are translucent. Add garlic, spices and herbs stirring constantly for another minute or so or until spices are very fragrant.
2. Add all vegetables (except chard) and remaining broth. Simmer with lid on for about 30 minutes or until vegetables are fork tender.
3. Remove 4 cups of soup and puree in a food processor. Add soup back to pot. Or, blend with immersion blender until the desired consistency is reached. Stir in Swiss chard and coconut milk. Reheat gently. Garnish with chopped basil or cilantro. For my vegetarian friends try a little melted asiago on top — crazy! After detox...

Detox or not — this is fabulous soup! A little more labor intensive, but well worth the effort.

Smokey Watermelon Gazpacho

8-10 Servings

8 cups of seedless watermelon, cut in small cubes

2 ripe tomatoes, chopped

3 tbsp extra virgin olive oil

1 yellow or orange bell pepper, diced

3 tbsp white balsamic vinegar or Bragg's apple cider vinegar

1 cucumber, peeled and diced

1-2 jalapenos, seeds removed and diced

1/2 cup diced purple onion

1/4 cup fresh lime juice (save zest for garnish)

2 garlic cloves, minced

1 cup mango or peach, peeled and chopped (fresh or frozen)

1 tsp smoked paprika

1/2 tsp ground chipotle pepper (or to taste)

1 1/2 tsp sea salt

2 tbsp fresh chopped basil

1/2 cup fresh chopped cilantro

Blend fruits, veggies, lime, vinegar and spices in large bowl. Use food processor or immersion blender to puree about two thirds of mixture. Stir in fresh herbs and cover tightly. Allow to chill in fridge for a few hours before serving. (This is way better the next day).

This Nature's Gatorade is always a huge hit at summer get togethers!

"When I was having that alphabet soup, I never thought that it would pay off" — Vanna White

Entrées and Sides to Nourish the Body & Soul

Mushrooms & Wilted Spinach with Wild Rice

4 Servings

---

1 tbsp olive oil

3 cups sliced assorted mushrooms

2 small shallots, minced

1-2 garlic cloves, minced

1 tsp fresh chopped thyme leaves (or 1/2 tsp dried)

1/4 cup dry white wine (after detox)

2 tsp Dijon mustard

1/4 cup water

3 cups spinach leaves (loosely packed)

2 cups prepared wild rice or quinoa

1. Over medium high heat add oil to large skillet (iron if you've got it). Throw in sliced shallots, dash of salt and mushrooms, sautéing for about 5 minutes. Add garlic and thyme. Sauté for another 5 minutes or so until mushrooms have released all their moisture.
2. Blend mustard with 1/4 cup water and set aside. Add wine to hot pan (after detox) and simmer for a minute or so to evaporate alcohol. Stir in mustard mix and bring to high simmer. Remove pan from heat. Toss in spinach and stir until wilted. Arrange on plate with a pretty mound of wild rice (I use a 1/2 cup stainless measuring cup as a mold for the rice). Garnish with fresh sprig of thyme and lemon wedge.

Who said suffering should be part of healthy eating. This recipe is no pain and all gain!

"If hunger makes you irritable — better to eat and be pleasant" — Sefer Hasidim

Orange and Ginger Glazed Beets on Top Fresh Spinach

4-6 Servings

---

1 lb beets, peeled and cubed (reserved beet greens for later)

1 cup fresh squeezed orange juice

2 tsp fresh grated ginger

4 drops organic liquid stevia (optional)

1/2 cup water

1 tbsp arrowroot or tapioca flour

4 cups of loosely packed fresh spinach

1. Combine beets, orange juice, ginger, stevia, and water in medium sauce pan. Bring to boil and reduce to simmer. Cook for about 15 minutes or until beets are fork tender.
2. Combine 1/4 cup of hot liquid from beets with arrowroot in small cup, whisking until arrowroot is completely dissolved. Slowly stir mixture into beets and simmer until sauce is just beginning to thicken.
3. Serve beets with a slotted spoon over fresh spinach and drizzle with sauce.

A beautiful dish hot or cold! These are not the canned beets you grew up with. Try it once and you'll be hooked on the purple passion!

I've converted many a beet hater. Use golden beets to fool the die – hard skeptic. TIP: Add prepared brown rice, wild rice or quinoa to your salad for a little added protein.

"One cannot think well, love well, sleep well, if one has not dined well" — Virginia Woolf

Quinoa and Roasted Brussels Stuffed Acorn Squash

4-6 Servings

Step 1: Ingredients

2 small acorn squash, halved with seeds discarded*

2 tsp olive oil

1 lb fresh Brussels sprouts, shredded

1/2 tsp dried thyme

1 tsp each of sea salt and cracked pepper

Step 2: Ingredients

1 cup quinoa (multi-color makes a beautiful presentation)

1 1/2 cup water or broth

2" piece of kombu, soaked in water until soft and then diced

Step 3: Ingredients

1 1/2 cup vegetable broth (reserve 1 cup)

2 leeks, chopped (white part with a little green — wash very well)

1 stalk of celery, chopped fine

2 garlic cloves, minced

1 tbsp rice flour or tapioca flour

1/4 cup white wine (or water)

1 tsp fresh thyme leaves, chopped

1 tsp cracked pepper

Roast Brussels sprouts

2 1/2 cups of prepared quinoa

Sea salt to taste

Step 1:

Pre-heat oven to 400°F. Rub flesh of each squash half with 1 tsp olive oil and sprinkle with salt and pepper. Place squash flesh side down on baking sheet. Toss Brussel sprouts in olive oil, salt, pepper and thyme. Spread evenly on another baking sheet. Bake Brussels and squash for 30 minutes or until tender. Note: Switch racks half way through for more even cooking.

Step 2:

Soak quinoa in cold water for 5 minutes. Rinse and drain through a fine mesh strainer. Bring water to boil in skillet or pan. Add quinoa and diced kombu. Bring back to boil and reduce to low simmer. Cook for 15 minutes uncovered or until water is completely absorbed. Remove from heat and set aside.

Step 3:

1. Heat large non-stick skillet over medium high and add 1/2 cup of broth. Add leeks and sauté for about 5 minutes, until leeks are soft. Add celery and garlic and sauté another few minutes.
2. Sprinkle flour over mixture and incorporate well, stirring constantly for just a minute to cook flour a little (do not burn). Add wine (after detox) or water to hot pan along with, fresh thyme and cracked pepper. Slowly add 1 cup of broth while stirring constantly. Bring to simmer until sauce is just thickening.
3. Fold in Brussels sprouts and quinoa. Add salt to taste. (TASTE FIRST!)

Stuff squash halves with quinoa mixture and garnish with a sprig of thyme. This is impressive!

*Butternut squash also works well.

Southern Style Collard Greens

4 Servings

---

1 tbsp olive oil

1/2 cup sliced onion

2 garlic cloves, minced

1 bunch of collard greens, stems removed and chopped*

1/2 cup water or vegetable broth

2 tsp red wine vinegar

Dash of sea salt and cracked pepper

In a large skillet, heat oil over medium high. Sauté onions with a dash of salt for about 3 minutes. Add garlic and sauté for a minute or so. Add collard greens and 1/2 cup of water or broth. Cover and simmer for 15-20 minutes, stirring occasionally until collards are tender. Uncover and stir in vinegar. Bring back to simmer for a few minutes until moisture is mostly evaporated. Add salt and pepper to taste.

*Save stems for soups

Steak & Mashed Potatoes — Not! With Garlicky Green Beans

4-6 Servings

Grilled Portobello Mushrooms

4 large Portobello mushrooms, wiped clean and stem removed

1 tbsp extra virgin olive oil

1 tbsp balsamic vinegar

1/2 tsp sea salt

cracked pepper to taste

Whisk oil, vinegar and seasonings together. Brush mushrooms with oil mixture on both sides and place gill side up in single layer in large glass dish. Allow to set in refrigerator covered for 1 hour.

Place mushrooms gill side up on hot grill. Grill for 4 to 5 minutes then flip. Grill for another few minutes. Watch closely — they burn easily!

Note: Mushrooms can also be broiled.

Cauliflower, Rutabaga & Garlic Smash

1 medium head of cauliflower, cut into florets

1 medium rutabaga, cubed

4-6 large garlic cloves, peeled and crushed

1 cup vegetable broth

1/4 cup nutritional yeast flakes*

Dash of cayenne

1/2 tsp cracked pepper (or to taste)

4 drops of organic liquid stevia (optional)

1 tbsp extra virgin olive oil

Sea salt and cracked pepper to taste

1. Place cauliflower, rutabaga, and garlic in steamer basket inside large pot. Add broth to pan, cover, and steam for about 20 minutes or until rutabaga is very tender. Drain off broth into cup or bowl and set aside.
2. Transfer steamed veggies to food processor. Add nutritional yeast, spices, stevia and olive oil. Process adding a little broth as needed until the consistency of whipped potatoes is reached (hand mixer works great too!).
3. Top with fresh chopped chives and a little cracked pepper.

*TIP: This protein rich miracle food has a rich buttery, cheesy flavor and is also a good source of vitamin B-12. It can be found at any natural foods store (in bulk or packaged).

Garlicky Cast Iron Green Beans

1/2 lb green beans, trimmed and blanched (or whole frozen beans thawed)*

2-3 garlic cloves, minced

1 tbsp olive oil

Sea salt and pepper to taste

1. Heat large cast iron skillet over medium high heat and add oil. Add garlic and then green beans, sautéing for a few minutes until crispy tender.
2. Add sea salt and cracked pepper to taste.

*Trim beans by snipping off the stem end. To blanch green beans just add them to a boiling pot of water for a minute or until they turn bright green. Remove with slotted spoon and plunge into ice bath to stop the cooking process. You can now cook or freeze your beans. This method works great for broccoli and asparagus as well.

A good meal soothes the soul as it regenerates the body. From the abundance of it flows a benign benevolence" — Frederick W. Hackwood

Braised Red Cabbage with Apples and Red Onions a top Sweet & Savory Smashed Turnips

4-6 Servings

---

*1-2" strip of kombu ***

1 tbsp avocado or sunflower oil

1 small head of red cabbage, cored and coarsely shredded

1 medium red onion, sliced thin

2 garlic cloves, minced

1/2 tsp caraway seed (optional)

2 small Granny Smith apples, cored and sliced thin

1/4 cup Bragg's apple cider vinegar

1/4 cup sweet white wine like Riesling (after detox), or 1/4 cup water

4 drops organic liquid stevia (optional)

Sea salt and cracked pepper to taste

1. Place kombu strip in water and set aside. Heat large skillet or wok over medium high heat. Add oil and swirl to coat skillet. Add onions, garlic, and caraway seeds (in that order) and sauté with a dash of salt for a few minutes.
2. Dice softened kombu and add it to skillet along with the balance of ingredients. Bring to boil and reduce to simmer. Cover and cook for about 20 or 30 minutes or until cabbage is tender, stirring occasionally. Add salt and pepper to taste.
3. Uncover and add wine or water. Bring to high simmer for a few minutes until most of liquid is evaporated.

Serve on top of Smashed Sweet and Savory Turnips. Garnish with fresh sprig of rosemary. This is the definition of comfort food!

*Kombu is a sea vegetable that packs a healthy punch of iodine and minerals. It's sweet and "non-fishy" making it compatible to a variety of dishes. It looks like green pepper or scallions when cooked — no one will ever know!

Smashed Sweet & Savory Turnips

2 lb turnips, peeled and cubed

4 drops organic liquid stevia

1 tsp coarse ground sea salt

1 sprig of rosemary or lavender (about 1")

Water for boiling

2 tsp extra virgin olive oil

1/4 cup nutritional yeast

1/4 cup canned coconut milk (or to desired consistency)

Sea salt and cracked pepper to taste

1. In large pot, add turnips, stevia, salt, rosemary and enough water to cover the turnips by 1". Bring to boil and reduce heat to high simmer. Cook turnips for about 20 minutes or until they are fork tender.
2. Drain water and remove rosemary sprig. Stir in olive oil, nutritional yeast and milk. Whip with electric mixer or by hand until creamy, adding milk a little at a time until desired consistency is reached.
3. Add cracked pepper and sea salt to taste. Garnish with a sprig of rosemary or lavender flower.

I loved these as much as mashed potatoes growing up! Most kids today don't know what they're missing.

What I say is that, if a man really likes potatoes, he must be a pretty decent sort of fellow." — A. A. Milne

Rosemary Infused Quinoa and Roasted Vegetables

4-6 Servings

---

1 cup quinoa

1 1/2 cup water or broth

1-2" sprig of rosemary

1 whole head of garlic

1 large sweet yellow onion, cut in half and quartered

1 red bell pepper, chopped into bite size chunks

1 carrot, sliced on diagonal about 1/4" thick

1 zucchini or yellow squash, sliced on diagonal about 1/4 thick

1 tsp olive oil

1 tsp sea salt and cracked pepper

1. Preheat oven to 400°F. Soak quinoa in cold water for 5 minutes. Rinse and drain through a fine mesh strainer. In large skillet or sauce pan, add quinoa, water and rosemary. Bring to boil and reduce to low simmer. Cook for 15 minutes uncovered or until water is completely absorbed. Remove from heat and set aside.
2. Cut tip off of garlic head to expose tops of cloves and remove outer layer of paper. In large bowl, toss garlic and vegetables in olive, salt and pepper. Spread onto baking pan. Bake for 15 to 20 minutes or until veggies are tender.
3. When cool enough to handle, holding root end of garlic head, squeeze out all the roasted cloves. Mince if desired. Toss garlic and roasted veggies together with quinoa and dressing (see below).

Dressing:

1 tbsp lemon juice

2 tbsp extra virgin olive oil

2 tbsp aged balsamic vinegar

1/4 cup nutritional yeast

1/2 tsp garlic salt

1/2 tsp onion powder

1 tbsp fresh chopped parsley (optional)

1/4 tsp red pepper flakes (or to taste)

Whisk all ingredients together until well blended, adding a little water if needed for thinner consistency.

"Food, like a loving touch or a glimpse of divine power, has that ability to comfort ." — Norman Kolpas

Easy Everyday Lentils

8 Servings

5 cups water or vegetable broth (reserve 1/4 cup)

1 onion, diced

1 stalk of celery, diced

3 cloves of garlic, minced

1 1/2 cups lentils, rinsed and drained

2" piece of kombu, soaked (reserve water)

Water as needed

Dressing

1 tbsp lemon juice

2 tbsp extra virgin olive oil

2 tbsp aged balsamic vinegar

1/4 cup nutritional yeast

1/2 tsp garlic salt

1/2 tsp onion powder

1 tbsp fresh chopped parsley (optional)

1/4 tsp red pepper flakes (or to taste)

A little water if needed for thinner consistency

1. Soak kombu in cup of water until soft (about 5 minutes). Set aside. Heat large sauce pan over medium high and add broth. Toss in onions and celery with a dash of salt. Sauté for a few minutes and add garlic, stirring for another minute or so.
2. Remove kombu from water and dice. Add soaking water and kombu to pan along with lentils and rest of broth. Bring to boil, reduce to simmer and cook with tilted lid, stirring occasionally for 20-30 minutes or until lentils are very tender. Add water as needed.

3. Whisk together all dressing ingredients and toss with lentils.

NOTE: Short on time? Leave out the sautéed vegetables and just add the dressing — still delicious and super easy! Be sure and make a double batch of dressing — great on salads too!

Lip Smackin' Smoothies!

Strawberries and Cream

1/2 cup frozen strawberries

1/2 cup fresh or frozen chopped rhubarb

6-8 ounces natural spring water

2 ounces canned coconut milk (coconut milk beverage if fat is an issue)

2 tbsp rice or hemp protein (no sugar added)

1 tsp flaxseed oil

1/4 tsp vanilla flavoring

4 drops of organic liquid stevia

Tropical Paradise

1/2 cup fresh or frozen pineapple

1/2 cup fresh or frozen mango

1/4 cup shredded carrots

6-8 ounces natural spring water

2 ounces canned coconut milk (coconut milk beverage if fat is an issue)

1/4 cup fresh chopped parsley

1 tsp flaxseed oil

2 tbsp rice or hemp protein (no sugar added)

1-2 drops organic liquid stevia

Orange Creamsicle

1 small orange or tangerine, peeled, seeded, and sectioned

1/2 frozen very ripe banana

6-8 ounces natural spring water

2 ounces canned coconut milk (coconut milk beverage if fat is an issue)

1/4 cup shredded carrots

1 tsp flaxseed oil

1/4 cup prepared plain quinoa

1-2 drops organic liquid stevia

1/2 tsp vanilla flavoring

Key Lime Pie

1/4 cup fresh squeezed lime juice

1/2 frozen ripe banana

6-8 ounces natural spring water

2 ounces canned coconut milk (coconut milk beverage if fat is an issue)

2 tbsp rice or hemp protein (no sugar added)

1/2 cup fresh or frozen spinach

1/4 cup fresh chopped parsley

1 tsp flaxseed oil

4 drops organic liquid stevia

1/4 tsp vanilla flavoring

1/4 tsp almond extract

Morning Mojito

1/4 cup fresh squeezed lime juice

1/4 cup fresh chopped parsley

2 tbsp fresh chopped mint

2 tbsp organic green powder (vegetables — NO SUGAR)

2 tbsp rice or hemp protein (NO SUGAR added)

6-8 ounces natural spring water

4 drops organic liquid stevia

Figs and Fennel & Fit as a Fiddle

3 large figs (fresh or frozen)

1/4 cup chopped fennel bulb

1/4 cup chopped cucumber (peeled or unpeeled)

1/2 cup chopped apple (peeled or unpeeled)

1/2 cup chopped kale

1 tsp flaxseed oil

Dash of nutmeg (optional)

6-8 ounces water

Blend all smoothies until fresh fruits and vegetables are pureed. Add water or ice for desired consistency.

Smoothie Tips:

Invest in a heavy duty blender.

Try using frozen fruit instead for a thicker, richer smoothie.

Bonus Recipes

Gail's Indian Brown Basmati Rice

6-8 Servings

---

2 tbsp coconut oil

1/2 cup chopped sweet onion

1 garlic clove, minced

1 cinnamon stick (2")

2-3 cardamom pods, split

2-3 whole cloves

1 tsp cumin seed

1 tsp ground turmeric

1 tsp sea salt

2 tbsp ground flaxseed

1 cup brown basmati rice

2 cups of water

1 cup diced carrots or parsnips

2" piece of soaked kombu

2 tbsp finely chopped celery leaves or 1/2 stalk celery, finely chopped

4 drops organic liquid stevia (use maple syrup after detox)

1/4 cup water

1. In large skillet with tight lid, melt coconut oil over medium high heat then reduce to medium. Add onions, garlic and a dash of salt. Sauté for a few minutes until onions are translucent and soft. Add spices and toast for a couple of minutes stirring constantly until fragrant. Add flaxseed and rice. Toast rice mixture for a couple of

minutes stirring often. Add water and bring to boil. Reduce to simmer and cover. Cook for 45 minutes and remove from heat immediately.

2. (Optional) While rice is cooking, place kombu in cup of water for about 5 minutes or until soft. Dice into small pieces. In small sauce pan, add kombu, carrots or parsnips, celery, stevia and water. Bring to boil and reduce heat to low simmer. Cover and cook for about 10 minutes or until carrots or parsnips are al dente (slightly crisp). Fluff rice with fork and toss with carrot mixture.

This rice is amazing hot or cold. Serve it in salads for a complete meal. Make a double batch for now and later — freezes beautifully!

Alkalizing Detox Lemonade

8 ounces natural spring water

4 drops organic liquid stevia

1-2 tsp Bragg's apple cider vinegar

Juice of 1 small lemon (organic juice in a jar works too — 1 TB)

Stir and enjoy hot or cold — fabulous! (Hint — vinegar neutralizes bitterness)

TIP: Use sparkling water for a soda substitute. Use fresh lime and 1 ounce of tart cherry juice (no sugar added) for an amazing cherry limeade!

Green Tea Lemonade with Fresh Mint and Stevia

10 regular green tea bags

12 cups purified water

1/4 cup of fresh stevia leaves

1/4 cup of fresh mint leaves

3 large lemons juiced (or 1/2 cup of juice)

2 tsp Bragg's apple cider vinegar

Organic liquid stevia to taste (optional)

In a 4-quart sauce pan, muddle mint and stevia leaves in a little lemon juice to release flavors. Add water, balance of lemon juice and tea bags. Bring to boil then remove pan from heat and steep tea with lid on for 4-6 minutes. Stir in vinegar and liquid stevia to taste. Strain tea into a large pitcher. Serve over ice and garnish with lemon wheel and sprig of mint. Delicious and soothing served warm.

Here's to your Peace, Joy, LOVE and Abundant Health!

Intuitive Chef Gail

About the Intuitive Chef

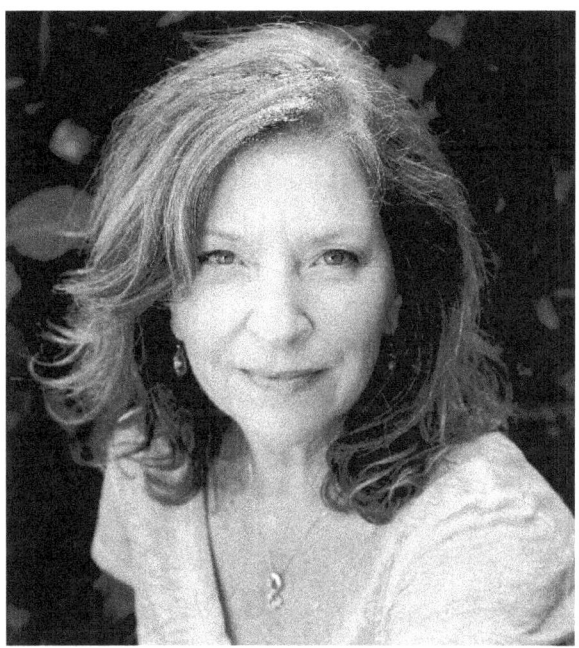

Gail's "Intuitive Chef" journey started unfolding in 2009 when she began working her passion creating delicious, nutritious food. What began as a true desire to help others enjoy abundant health through the power of food, led her down an unexpected and wondrous path of "awakening".

As a plant-based chef turned Food & Medical Intuitive in 2012 she has helped thousands all over the world remember their natural, God-given health through her "Food IS Talking" Intuitive Food Compatibility process. The food charts reveal to her what the client's body wants to eat to restore balance (the first step to healing), to detox and to move it into thrive mode. This intuitive approach is unique to every "body" and reveals as well, the state of the body at any given time.

Over the years, as her gifts have expanded, she has become a conduit for "revelation", the name she gives to the Divine Wisdom and Guidance she receives. 7 vitally important revelations regarding health and well-being were received over a 7 year period. These revelations led her to begin creating the Evolution of FREE Health workshops, books and video series.

The first book, **The Quinoa Cookbook Journey** is a super creative and tasty introduction to the series. There are 2 more books in this series to be released in 2023. Stay tuned for **The 7 Missing Links to Abundant & Sustainable Health** and **Commanding Your Vessel**.

Latest Workshop Offerings:

Evolution of Free Health Workshop:
Become your own Food Intuitive

A Course in Discernment:
Mastering Divine Discernment/The Truth is Written Within

Keep up with Gail at:

foodrevelation.com
facebook.com/foodrevelation
facebook.com/evolutionoffreehealth
twitter.com/foodrevelation
youtube.com/channel/UCWT8yh9wQfMR6gu79P1KfXw

Gail works remotely with clients all over the world. Schedule a no-charge 15 minute exploratory session here:
foodrevelation.com/schedule

Disclaimer: I am not a doctor or licensed nutritionist. I am an intuitive. Services and information provided in the form of tips, recipes, and nutrition advice does not qualify as a substitution for your medical doctor's protocol or advice. I encourage you to trust your instincts and do what feels right to you, but seek guidance from your doctor concerning your health and wellness.

www.ingramcontent.com/pod-product-compliance
Lightning Source LLC
Chambersburg PA
CBHW060353130626
46553CB00003B/1211